THE ROCKY ROAD OF 24/7

SYLVIA'S UPS AND DOWNS AND POSITIVE
LEARNINGS ALONG THE WAY (NEW EDITION)

Sylvia Bryden-Stock

Author's Tranquility Press
Marietta, Georgia

Copyright © 2022 by Slyvia Bryden-Stock.

All rights reserved. No part of this publication may be reproduced, distributed or transmitted in any form or by any means, including photocopying, recording, or other electronic or mechanical methods, without the prior written permission of the publisher, except in the case of brief quotations embodied in critical reviews and certain other noncommercial uses permitted by copyright law. For permission requests, write to the publisher, addressed "Attention: Permissions Coordinator," at the address below.

Slyvia Bryden-Stock/Author's Tranquility Press
2706 Station Club Drive SW
Marietta, GA 30060
www.authorstranquilitypress.com

Ordering Information:
Quantity sales. Special discounts are available on quantity purchases by corporations, associations, and others. For details, contact the "Special Sales Department" at the address above.

THE ROCKY ROAD OF 24/7/ Slyvia Bryden-Stock
Paperback: 978-1-957208-89-3
eBook: 978-1-957208-90-9

CONTENTS

ACKNOWLEDGMENTS 1
FOREWORD 2
INTRODUCTION 5
WE NEVER THOUGHT 10
SETTLING IN TACTICS – SEEING IT THROUGH 15
A CHRISTMAS DILEMMA DESTINED TO BE A GREAT TEACHER 23
SELF CARE AND "WHERE'S MY MONEY!" 33
SELF-UNDERSTANDING AND CO-OPERATION 39
KEEPING A SENSE OF HUMOUR 45
LOSING IT ALL DOWN THERE!! 52
IT WOULD HAVE TO BE MY HUSBAND 59
FOOD GLORIOUS FOOD 68
BE READY FOR SUPRISES! 75
THE DUMMY RUN AND IT'S OUTCOMES 82
A SUMMARY OF LITTLE TIPS 92
ABOUT THE AUTHOR 94

ACKNOWLEDGMENTS

To my very special husband who through his journey has been a key part in helping to develop coaching and other tools to bring some light to what is a very different emotional journey for careers.

To my dear friend Angela who has edited this book for me as well being a wonderful support throughout.

To my sister, other family members and friends who also have supported us both on our journey thus far.

To Princess Christian Care Home who give loving, patient care at a very high standard.

To the all-knowing universal power that has been my inner anchor through difficult moments

FOREWORD

As the owner of Nursing Homes, I meet people in what is often the most challenging time of their lives, whether it is a resident with Dementia or a relative caring for the person.

I know that no-one aspires to being admitted into a Dementia Nursing Home as they live their journey.

Yet the people that work there and the relatives that are involved, do so with huge compassion, bravery, determination and love.

They can make a huge difference by working together to overcome the challenges, but it can take a huge toll emotionally.

Sylvia's books are not only a huge help for anyone going through the trauma of losing a loved one to Dementia, but also a valediction of love's little victories casting light into the darkest of times.

Sylvia is special – She has thrown herself into her husband's care with all she has and I wish everyone had a Sylvia to support them. Brian's journey is brighter because of her.

Nevertheless, my role has taught me that everyone is special!

We can all make a difference and you don't have to do it alone.

The previous book "The Rocky Road of Naughty Neurons" is equally inspiring as it expresses the challenges faced leading up to the Nursing Home journey.

I urge you to not only read her books – But feel them.

With love,
Martin Barrett
Managing Director
Nellsar Ltd

"Life doesn't require that we be the best, only that we try our best."

- Jackson Brown Jr.

INTRODUCTION

I never thought for one moment that my life purpose was to come from the journey I am still on as I write this book.

My past career as a nurse, working for many years in the community brought me into close contact with patients and families on journeys with terminal disease, chronic conditions as well as the Dementia arena.

It taught me a lot about the day-to-day challenges that both patient and family careers go through as they try to cope with the ever worsening of their loved ones condition taking place 24/7 right in front of their eyes.

I watched as beautiful living rooms changed from places of companionship, celebration, and fun events were turned into a clinical setting with hospital bed, wheelchair, hoist and commode adorning the once, perhaps, opulent surroundings. The beautiful dining table was shrouded with boxes of vinyl gloves, syringes, wound dressing packs, packs of incontinence pads and other medically related items including an array of drugs in a specially designed "dosset box" – the term for a safe container for drugs. The continuous hum of the pressure sore prevention mattress motor became the background sound behind the television programs. In amongst this and the frequent, essential visits from nurses and careers, a semblance of normal living was attempted.

One could not help becoming quite an integral part of that setting plus the emotions expressed or suppressed by the family and friends involved.

Some years later, I found myself working as a Care Home Manager, coming face to face with all the dynamics that are part of the caring environment –

Maintaining a happy team of staff

Ensuring Residents were well cared for

Keeping relatives up to date with their loved ones care, as well as being counsellor and comforter in times of great stress or the frustration of being a support and career to their loved one.

Meeting required standards and ensuring Senior Management could see a profitable organisation.

There are good days and not so good days.

I recall one of the key Sisters in charge on a typical morning shift, greeting me as I entered the home. She would rush to greet me and almost joyously declare "Matron we have SO many Problems today!" By now, heavily into personal growth strategies I would respond with "We don't have problems in this home – we have challenges that we face up to and deal with.!" A look and a shake of the head would communicate that she was more than capable of Dealing with the day-to-day niggles on her shift and a short discussion reinforced it as I used encouraging and empowering strategies. Later on, I would have a report of the successes achieved!

Doesn't life have challenges from day to day anyway? It is all about how they are faced up to.

Then there was a relative who insisted that her mother always wore the very best of Jaeger clothing that money could buy. Then what happened? A well - meaning night duty carer decide to help with the laundry. The resident concerned had a beautiful wool and cashmere Jaeger jumper that was in the washing pile. She put the jumper in a washing machine with clothes on a fairly hot wash that would tolerate the temperature and then tumble dried it!!

Matron, of course drew the short straw to show the daughter a jumper that was no longer adult size but would fit a three-year-old!! (This had happened before my time, I found out later). As daughter was not providing practical and quality clothing for mother to look great in, all staff breathed a sigh of relief when she arrived with a large washing basket and sign to alert everyone that she would take mothers washing and do it herself.

I have to say this incident helped with my choice of clothing for my husband that was both practical but allowed him to maintain his always well co-ordinated look.

Fast forward to my agency nursing to help maintain income levels. Care Homes of all shapes and sizes were now my work territory, working both day and night shifts. This was a very interesting experience I witnessed superb standards and not so good standards of overall care even though most of the staff were coming from a "heart centered" work ethic.

Time passes and I am more heavily weighted with my holistic and spiritual endeavors plus the man in my life is loving me unconditionally for who I am and who I need to become – I am truly blessed! He had his own barn dance band and was a great folk singer. We had So many fun times together.

Never in a million years did I expect to wake up one day having to accept a journey of Young Onset Alzheimer's Disease. I had witnessed Alzheimer's and other Dementia related diseases needing carer input, never dreaming that one day that would be me!

In the previous book, "The Rocky Road of Naughty Neurons", I take you from pre-diagnosis days to early care home days.

This book takes you on an insightful path of what it is like to be a career when your loved one is now in 24/7 care in a care home.

Come with me now as I share pains, learnings and laughter plus inner growth experiences that ultimately have led to a major part of my life purpose playing out to help others on their caring journey with Alzheimer's Disease. There may be some repetition throughout that is designed to help you as you travel on your own journey.

CHAPTER 1

WE NEVER THOUGHT

A typical day in the life of a career and her husband in the very early stages of their journey, today is the monthly meet-up at the Working Alzheimer's Society Day Centre where careers and those diagnosed indulge in coffee and biscuits, open chat, plus a sharing of ideas and challenges, followed by a buffet lunch.

The early morning of my husband getting dressed has gone relatively smoothly without too many frustration expletives flying around.

"It's the lunch and social get together today darling" I say with deliberate excitement.

"I'm not going to that f…..g place! You can go on your own if you like!" he retorts with is Alzheimer's neurons language as well as his own frustration with things in his life now.

"Yes, but you will enjoy it when we get there. They put on free coffee and lunch every time!"

The mention of free food and coffee seemed to work and I managed to get him out the front door and into the car successfully. The Alzheimer's neurons soon kicked in again as we drive to the venue "Hm! I know where you're taking me!" he grumpily expresses. Deciding it was best to say nothing I remained silent and continued to drive the last little bit to the building. Luckily the drive was only about ten minutes from door to door. Thankfully there is a parking space close to the entrance. I press the entry buzzer and a familiar face appears moving towards the door to let us in. "Hello Brian" she says with a smile that says "I am pleased to see you" "It's lovely to see you again. Wow! You are looking smart as always. Come on in and have a cup of coffee and biscuits." The offer of coffee and biscuits seems to change his mood and before long his gregarious nature takes over and he is in full flow of conversation and laughing just like he always used to be. Yes! A very different man to the one earlier!!

I can now relax and join in the conversation as well as interact with the other careers. Lunch was a bit of a challenge for myself as I have a wheat and dairy intolerance and the table is set with French bread, butter and cheeses along with cakes that were out of bounds for me - jam and iced doughnuts that of course Brian indulged in! I took a plate and made a few crisps and grapes look really filling, along with indulging in some fruit juice, and accepted that at least they were healthy plus the fact that Brian was obviously having a good time. It was far better to focus on the joyous moments here than the challenge of actually getting him to attend.

Now – a very interesting thing happened on this particular day. One couple who we became good friends with were talking about a relative who was in a local care home and were praising the home highly. It was a Care Home I had not heard of before – Princess Christian Care home in Bisley, Surrey. "I've never heard of that one" I commented "I know many locally from my past experience but not this one. Where exactly is it?" They gave me the address and having an inquisitive spirit, I said to Brian "I would love to go and see that home out of curiosity." He was, right at that moment, his old unconditional self and was happy to visit the care home.

The care home setting was down a quiet lane/bridleway with a fairly large car park and well looked after frontage. The actual building was of modern design but when I checked the internet later, I found it had quite a history to it.

Lord Roberts and Princess Christian, daughter of Queen Victoria had lost a son in the Boer war (1899-1902) and they both wanted to help young men coming back from Africa. At the time Homes for wounded soldiers were a novel concept but the public quickly supported and donations were made. Lord Pirbright donated some of his land to the incorporated Soldiers and Sailors Help Society and

Lord Roberts Workshops, and so four separate homes were built in 1902. The name derives from the president at that time — Princess Christian. The Princess Christian Home was designed to be a home of rest for discharged servicemen.

In 1997 the home was closed and the land left to become derelict. In 2005 Nelsar Homes bought the site and major renovation took place, with an opening in 2009 as a residential and nursing home for elderly and dementia residents.

The Care Home Manager was in reception when we walked in and had a very friendly and calm energy about him. I told him of the main reason for visiting and we found ourselves openly talking of Brian's recent diagnosis. As we chatted in the cosy visitor's room, I sensed that he managed the home from a heart centred approach. "Would you like to have a look round?" he asked. "Is that OK with you Brian?" I felt that was the right thing to do, especially as we had our plan for doing this journey totally at home. "Sure" was his response.

The first thing that struck me about the home was the pristine cleanliness of the place and the total lack of a smell of urine. As is said in the profession — it passed the nose test! The rooms were a good size and the corridors had bright coloured decorative collage borders and pictures that created a homely ambience within the required setting for care. With a large garden area at the rear plus patios outside the lounges and conservatories, the home for me came up trumps.

Now, here's the thing folks! As we are walking around the care home Brian turns to the manager and says in a distinct voice "You know – if ever I have to have care in a care home, I would be happy to come here!" Mentally I was shocked to hear those words and said nothing. Especially as, for me, the visit was out of pure curiosity and the "do it at home" plan was firmly fixed with me at that time. I had no intention of "dumping" my lovely man in a care home! We left with a brochure and the manager gave me his business card and said that I could contact him at any time.

Off home we went and I did my best to "be in the moment" and keep life as "normal" as possible. The brochure was filed away and no more was said. Especially as we both had agreed on our plan for this journey of ours.

Now – fast forward to 2014 …………

CHAPTER 2

SETTLING IN TACTICS – SEEING IT THROUGH

By now my husband is actually having day care at Princess Christian Care Home and in spite of challenges to get him there, he enjoys the day and is all smiles when I pick him up. We had tried the day centre at the local Alzheimer's Society but he didn't enjoy the format so having had to take respite care at Princess Christian Care Home (see The Rocky Road of Naughty Neurons), it made sense to organize day care at the same place.

The days and nights were becoming more challenging for myself as his "naughty neurons" kicked in more and more. Angry outbursts resulted in the living room curtains being pulled down plus punching me from time to time. Add to that the major sundowning with little or no sleep at all plus his absolute refusal to have care input at home I was becoming aware of the challenge facing me of letting go some more was drawing closer. The emotions around facing a further decision were overwhelming. However, I continued to call on my inner "higher self" strength and use the mantra "I choose Peace – All is Well in my World"

After a week of exacerbated Alzheimer's behaviour, the day dawned for his Thursday day care in November of 2014. I had jokingly had a chat with the receptionist at Princess Christian on the Monday not thinking that it might be shared with the Care Home Manager! Strangely I found myself saying, almost as a prayer, on the Thursday morning as we went through the now "more interesting" routine of assisted washing and dressing "If I have to make a decision about Brian's ongoing care then the Manager will be in the reception area when we arrive.

Oh my! As we entered the Care Home who should be waiting to greet us but the Manager! My stomach churned as the fateful words hit my ears–

"Sylvia, why don't you bring a few of Brian's clothes later on and let him stay?" My prayer had been answered and not totally as I wanted but deep down, I knew it was the right one. With a smiling face, I left my darling man who I loved deeply and unconditionally, and drove home sobbing as I expressed my human emotions about the next phase on this journey I was travelling. I called a friend of ours who has known us for many years and facilitated our wedding blessing service. She had said from the start of our journey

"I am here for you Sylvia at Any Time" How blessed we were to have such a friend.

When I called her, she was at home and through tears I shared what was happening. In minutes she was at the house and I released the pain of the journey as she said a prayer. I then began to become calm and find a sense of inner peace. "She truly is a blessing and a true friend" I thought after she left. I sent up a prayer of thanks and knew deep down that I would face this next phase of the journey building even greater inner strength and peace; that I would acknowledge moments of sadness and pain and turn them into positive outcomes to help others as we had both vowed at the very beginning.

Doing my best to stay calm, I went upstairs and packed some clothes and personal care items to take to the care home. "What am I going to say to hm?". The question kept echoing through my mind as I almost robotically seemed to be getting his things together.

I thought back to my time as a Care Home Manager when I would deal with this situation from "the other side of the fence" as it were. The relatives would be coached as to the best way they could help their loved one settle in. "It will best not to visit every day – even have a week without visiting." They are in good care and we will look after them. You can phone at any time to get an update from us". Then there was advice about letting their loved one understand they needed an assessment and monitoring to establish the best form of care. I never thought for a minute it would one day be me!!

I decided that my way of dealing with this moment would be to focus on his "sundowning" behavior and tell him he had been advised to have a sleep assessment to help sort it out.

Next, I made myself some lunch as I knew I needed to keep my strength up and care for me as best I could.

The old guilt feelings emerged as I realised that my/our original plan had been totally abandoned and there was no turning back. Yet deep down inside there was the awareness of knowing that change does not have to be accepted through guilt – beating oneself up for perceiving you are a failure.

In the house I have **a plaque that belonged to my mother that states** –

God Grant Me The Serenity

To Accept the Things I Cannot Change

To Change the Things I Can

And The Wisdom to Know The Difference

- Anonymous

You see, in life, you cannot always change the circumstances but you can change the way you look at them and make a decision that empowers you to go through whatever it is and learn from it.

Late afternoon I went back to the care home and gave a staff member his things for his room. At the same time, I was given a web site called Snappy Tags to order some small clip-on labels that are discreet and not outwardly visible. They can be ordered and sent directly to the home. This saves a lot of time ordering and then sewing on labels for any new clothing. Then I went back to his unit and told him as best I could without showing emotions that it had been advised that he stay for a time to have his sleep issues assessed and monitored. He seemed to accept this which was a relief and I courageously left him before supper. The feelings I experienced were a combination of sadness that it had come to a point of 24/7 care coupled with some relief that I could now catch up on some well needed sleep!

My first night alone was somewhat restless as I began to come to terms with "this is it now Sylvia; he is into a new phase of his Alzheimer's journey". One thing I was pleased about was the fact that he was in an amazing place that had heart centred leadership and heart centred staff.

There was no way I could stay away the following day so I went to see him and he seemed cheery enough and still in acceptance of having to stay for a while. Part of me wanted to believe that I was living a lie but another part of me knew that this was the best tactic to use as part of his adjustment period.

After a couple of days, I took his washing home and left some new clean ones – thankfully he had always been a man with an extensive wardrobe. It felt good to be doing his washing and ironing as I had been doing before and I gained a degree of comfort from it.

About a week to ten days had passed and I was in his room collecting more washing when one of the male carers appeared in the doorway. "Sylvia, why are you taking Brian's washing home? He gently and caringly asked "We do that here for you. Leave them with me and I will take them to the laundry for you. I know this is a difficult time for you but let us help you and we will take good care of him. He will have everything that he needs." As I handed him the carrier bag of clothes, the stark reality of what was happening hit home again. Yes, a few more tears were shed as I left, but, once again, deep down I knew I had to be strong and learn new things that would turn into experiences to help other relatives on their own journey.

I visited most days and was greeted with a big hug and a kiss plus he appeared to be in good spirits. After a couple of weeks, the staff reported that he was interacting with other relatives as well as the staff and he was fast becoming "Mr. Popular on the unit!" He always was a very gregarious man which had made him successful in sales, plus, of course, the popularity of his Barn Dance Band called Stock Brokers Belt.

As the weeks went by, he was beginning to realise that I was not taking him home. I would be greeted with "It must be time for me to come home now!" As best I could I lovingly explained that until the doctor had got to the bottom of his sleep issues he would have to stay. Then I would change the conversation and keep it as lighthearted as possible to distract from his obvious frustration of having to be where he was.

My best comfort during this time was that the staff from Manger downward had a wonderful way of helping new residents settle in. They would appoint one member of staff to be with them to help create confidence and trust as now it was a "stranger" who would assist with personal care. For a man who was both independent and meticulous with his personal care and appearance this would be a major hurdle during the settling in period. Of course, he was encouraged to do as much as he could for himself including going to the toilet and being prepared for "Percy to miss the porcelain"! The patience I witnessed from the carers and nurses was incredible. With a whole unit of residents to be washed and dressed each morning, I did feel for them in respect of the time it would take with my husband to "assist" with his washing and dressing.

I made a point of typing out a typical day at home just prior to admission, with his likes and dislikes at that time along with how much assistance was required with personal care and eating which were impacted by not only his Alzheimer's neurons but also his Posterior Cortex Atrophy - gradual deterioration of the part of the brain that interprets what our eyes send through and we then can see.

As the days and weeks passed, I could see him beginning to show signs of adapting to his new environment and thought back to the day we visited out of pure curiosity on my part, and his words to the Manager "Well, if ever I need to go into a care home, I would be happy to come here". It was almost as if he was predicting his own future!

Gradually I was adjusting to dealing with his "It must be time to come home now!" I reassured him that I was taking care of the house and that all his money was safe and nobody else could touch it without our say so – thank goodness we arranged Power of Attorney when he had full mental capacity.

He got on exceedingly well with the manager Mario and I often witnessed them having a chat and laughing together when I visited.

Before I knew it Christmas was looming and I had to handle the issue of us having Christmas at the Care Home. Here lies another learning curve

....

CHAPTER 3

A CHRISTMAS DILEMMA DESTINED TO BE A GREAT TEACHER

December sees lots of pre-Christmas activity in the care home environment and Princess Christian was in full swing to make sure the residents, relatives and staff all has a great time during the festive season.

Reception was adorned with a stunningly decorated Christmas tree from floor to ceiling and the Christmas raffle tickets were selling well. Prizes had been donated by local enterprises wanting to support such a high standard care home. I indulged in some raffle tickets early in the month and made sure they were safely stored in a place where I would easily remember where they were.

The main event of the month was the Christmas party so I made sure that nothing else clashed with that day as it seemed important to me that the home was supported and Brian was encouraged to join in as many activities as possible. His favourite was when a singer came to entertain due to his love of music plus having been a great folk singer himself.

As Christmas drew closer, I was mentally planning how I would approach it with hm as it would be only six weeks following his admission along with his frequent request about coming home. I decided on what I felt was a sensitive approach rather than tell him he was not coming home for Christmas and provoke a typical "naughty neurons" outburst. "Leave it till it is really close to Christmas" I thought. The last few Christmases had been spent quietly together watching films which he really enjoyed – no hassle just the two of us together which would also minimize any outbursts due to frustration and a lot of noise. As I penned this chapter in a notebook before typing with quotes on some of the pages, my eyes were drawn to a lovely quote which seems very apt. I will now share it with you –

"When faced with a dilemma, take a moment to sit with the issue. Don't rush to decide what to do. Intend to let Divine inspiration flow to you, and it will be so."

Christine Northrup

This quote is a wonderful message for carers as well as in life generally. Another phrase I have heard over the years comes to mind - "put brain into gear before you open your mouth!" I was determined to have brain in gear before I broached the subject of where we would spend Christmas.

The care home Christmas party was the week prior to Christmas and I worked on getting my man to attend. There were two main ingredients to success –

- The very talented male singer who had been booked
- Festive food in abundance would be served late pm.

They worked!! He was definitely up for it!!

Party day dawns and as the morning progressed the housekeeping and activities teams along with the kitchen staff were in full swing converting the adjoining unit into a festive area complete with a tombola stall lovingly prepared by a relative. She put a lot of hard work into this – stuffing pieces of drinking straws with rolled up raffle tickets and sticking tickets number a 5 or 0 at the end on lots of bottles and other prizes. The care staff got SO excited when tombola stalls appeared and would spend a lot of their hard-earned cash on "having a go" to get a 5 or 0 ticket and win a prize! When success was reached a loud cheer rang out in the unit as they shared their success with each other. It was a great fund raiser for the home as relatives plus residents with full mental capacity joined in as well. My first attempt at tombola was not a success but at least I felt I was helping a good cause. These monies helped fund extras for the home that were not necessarily within the restraints of the annual budget.

The festive mood was very apparent with a staff member dressed up as Santa Claus. He approached Brian with "Have you been good this year? If you have, I shall be visiting you at Christmas." The responsive look said it all!! Not impressed! However, the singer came up trumps for him as he clapped and whooped shouting "More!" as well as joining in popular songs he could still recall with either vocals or a whistle. For me it was a joy to see him happy and relaxed, having fun. His veracious appetite was well and truly satisfied when the festive food was served. Now, here's the thing folks – on returning to his unit he was, for sure, ready to tuck into supper that was being served.

I decided to make my departure after supper with awareness of maybe having to deal with that question again "Isn't it time for me to come home?". He mentioned that he was missing me and I responded lovingly about my own feelings whilst managing to keep my cool. Emotions were best dealt with away from the care home environment.

Emphasizing that they were still having difficulty with sorting out his night time challenges was a regular visiting tactic, and the challenge of not visiting daily still brought up emotions but I knew that inner courage would build to help face the new journey that was taking place.

As Christmas got closer and closer, I decided to suggest that we had lunch at the Care Home as they were doing it "free" and would be able to cater for my dietary requirements. It was about five days before Christmas and I literally prayed for a sign that I could broach the Christmas Day/Boxing Day subject. Sure enough Brian asked me what we were doing for Christmas. "Why don't we spend Christmas day here?" I suggested "They will put on a wonderful spread and it will not cost us anything." Of course, I knew that there would be a donation required of me for that day but it was better to be shrewd about things as part of the ongoing adjustment to permanent stay. I breathed a sigh of relief when he agreed. If I was to take him home over the Christmas period, he would think he was staying home forever! No, that was definitely NOT an option! I know some of you reading this may disagree with my tactics at this point but this is where my own experience as a care home manger comes in to play. It is critical to prevent confusion and excessive agitation as they get used to their new environment and new daily routine. I was frequently reassured of Brian's integration with the staff and residents with no signs of visible depression or being unhappy.

One major thing that helped me in the early days following his admission was drawing on my inner spiritual strength and determination to find a way to create ongoing inner peace. I do believe that deep within everyone is a wonderful presence that will help if we seek it.

The other thing that gave me courage was looking back at the day when we did the "nosiness" visit and Brian stated that he would be happy to go into Princess Christian Care Home if ever he needed care. That was such a blessing to me!

Well, here we are and Christmas Day has dawned. I woke to my first Christmas day without turning over to wish my man a happy Christmas. Emotions welled up within me but I made a conscious choice to not dwell on them but get ready for a day with him at the care home. For a number of years, we had chosen not to buy each other gifts, just a loving card as neither of us had any great "wants" that could not be bought during the year. This made it easier under the current circumstances.

We had exchanged cards on Christmas Eve on my short visit. The staff had assisted him with signing a card – I bought one that said what I knew he would want to say. It had been sneaked in one day to the activities team and they took over! Interestingly, his non questioning about how the card manifested told me where he was on his journey. Due to the Posterior Cortex Atrophy along with dexterity issues, he was very challenged with writing but the staff were patient with him and I actually received the card from him with his name in it and some kisses that were penned by him with some assistance. It is now with my collection of cards from him that I treasure.

My belief is that we should carry out "normal" life patterns as much as we can during the early stages and not assume that they cannot understand us or participate in events and activities. Moments of clarity can easily catch us out and get us into trouble if we are not prepared for them.

I dressed in festive style on Christmas day and arrived at the care home at around 11am in time for a Christmas sing-along in my husband's unit. I joined in the singing and Brian sat quietly watching. I couldn't help but wonder in my mind what was going through his own mind, now somewhat confused with the "naughty neurons" activity. Before lunch was served, I had a great idea!!?? I took Brian into the visitor's room in the reception area, and made calls to family members from my iPhone and he had a chance to chat with them. I felt good about what I had done to help his overall Christmas experience as we went back into his unit and headed to the dining room for lunch. Tables were adorned with crackers and flowers plus sherry and wine glasses for those able to indulge in a little alcohol. The sound of the crackers being pulled seemed to exacerbate Brian's sound hypersensitivity so we did not pull our crackers but gently dismantled them to find our hat, toy and silly joke!

All was going well apart from him being somewhat quiet. Was he confused as to why we were not together at home? Then it happened!!!

He threw his cutlery down on to his plate, got up and very loudly with a few "f" words thrown in, began a tirade of abuse and stormed out of the dining room and into the far lounge. My instinct told me that it was best to let the staff deal with him as he was extremely agitated and angry and I could have been on the receiving end of his "naughty neurons" anger! "Are you alright Sylvia?" kind relatives asked "yes, I am fine thank you" I responded politely, hiding the inner pain inside.

The realisation then dawned on me! My great idea of the phone calls probably triggered the confusion around Christmas at the Care Home that created the unfortunate outburst. It was also a reminder that he was probably further on with his journey than was overtly obvious.

A major lesson was again learned about the integration period of our loved one into their "new home". You cannot necessarily create a smooth ride on this part but learn from the situations that crop up. One might also say that this is where it is so important to be aware of how you react as the carer and seek to create that inner calm and do your best to "observe" before jumping in with what might seem "a good idea"!

After finishing my own lunch, I kept out of his way for a while to allow him to calm down. We had afternoon tea and Christmas cake together before I left and returned home to reflect and deal with my "guilt" over the choice I had made about calling family members. After some tears and remorse, I realised that, yes, it was a major lesson learned and that I would be extra sensitive towards visits over the coming weeks until he realised that Princess Christian was his new home.

One major hurdle, as a carer facing the care home journey, which has to be faced up to, is accepting that this is a whole different ball game and emotions may well run high, especially in the early days. It can be all too easy to begin projecting ones own guilt and denial of what is happening on to others, even the staff at the care home. Life itself can create inner guilt which is turned into criticism of others instead of facing ones own feelings and letting go old patterns of guilt that usually come from a past experience, even as far back as childhood. One looks for ways to cover up guilt and denial issues going on inside.

As I began this new phase of my own journey as a carer, I knew that I had to face up to whatever the experience brought about and let go the guilt that seemed to rear its ugly head again – "Why couldn't I do this at home?" Stepping back to be the observer of the situation enabled me to see the reality of how my husband's neurons were impacting on his behavior. Certainly, the Christmas Day episode enabled me to face both guilt and denial and vow to respond from a new understanding. I consciously made a pact with myself to always look for the best in what was taking place with his care. Acknowledging that there would be times when his behavior would challenge the staff. That they would deal with it in a way that minimized outbursts as well as protecting themselves.

So, Christmas and Boxing Days survived, I had a day without visiting and tried to relax and draw on my "inner strength" for the next visit which began yet another phase on our journey ……….

CHAPTER 4

SELF CARE AND "WHERE'S MY MONEY!"

As I look Back to those early days, I realise the importance of ongoing acceptance plus creating balance in life as much as possible. Acknowledging that a fairy godmother isn't going to wave her magic wand and take life back to what it used to be. The best plan of action is to practice recalling happy times and face the challenges that lie ahead; taking one day at a time or even better, one moment at a time.

Way back in the early days when Brian had a good degree of mental capacity, and was able to make rational decisions, we set up Power of Attorney with myself as the key person with responsibility. Regarding this, from our experience, it makes sense to set up power of attorney for both finances and health when one is fit and well, keeping it in a safe place in case it is needed later on. It can prevent the potential for family feuds and disagreements. Sadly, these can arise – my community nursing days showed me some "interesting" scenarios that I did not want to live through myself if at all possible.

Well, speaking of finances and Power of Attorney, my next visit to the care home was not quite what I expected. A visit had transpired by those who were not happy about our wedding (see The Rocky Road of Naughty Neurons) that seemed to have had an impact on Brian. As soon as I walked in, I noticed he looked somewhat angry and, before I could even say hello, he roared at me "Where's my money?". It took me some time to reassure him. He remembered in a confused way, the visit, and whatever transpired left him very concerned about money issues. My approach was to calmly listen and then reassure him that all money was safe and that I was looking after it plus no-one could just take his money. By now it was afternoon tea time with cake, fruit and cups of tea – including his new taste for two teaspoons of sugar - being served. Thankfully this was a perfect distraction! The money episode did rear its ugly head from time to time for a while, but I was able to face it with a calm spirit and ignore the butterflies in my tummy that were still a part of the visiting events.

Conversations with the care staff and activities team revealed that overall, Brian was settling in and getting on well with all the staff. His gregarious nature and charm were still very evident at this stage. Any frustration and anger seemed to come in my direction! Do you remember the song of many years ago? – "You always hurt the one you love". Boy was that true at this stage, albeit it was more that his naughty neurons and confused frustration that created his outbursts. Maybe my blessing is that I have a fairly patient nature plus my nursing and care background, along with coaching skills to come into play on our journey. I do believe we cope with life better when we see our glass as half full rather than half empty. The issue of money came up from time to time under different guises. I was thankful again for past experience, new learnings, and some guidance from the staff.

"Who pays for all the food and things?" I would be asked on repeated occasions. The worst thing I could have said was that his money was paying for it all! Suffice it to say, I know what his response would have been, involving denial of ever agreeing to me overseeing money issues. Yes, those forgetful Alzheimer's Neurons!

And so it was, he accepted that it was the care home that provided all the things he needed with the manager seeing to it that everything was taken care of for him. Dealing with Alzheimer's symptoms requires much sensitivity around communication – and yes, sometimes you might feel that you are "living a lie". Yet, in a sense, it is better to be creative with the truth to ease the situation. You must judge for yourself and deal with any reactions that occur with a calm spirit. Arguments on this journey do not solve anything – only exacerbate the situation. For me arguments in life don't serve a great purpose. Discussion and valuing differences work far better. Let's face it. We all have our view of life and the world and differences should be a positive stimulating experience for us all. What comes to mind as I write is something I recall from the Bible that states in the book of Proverbs in the Old Testament – "A soft answer turneth away wrath". Of course, I realise that it may not always work on this journey, so the next best thing to do is walk away and allow them to be distracted by the staff – more on that later.

So, it is now into the New Year of 2015 and I am visiting as often as I can. A wake-up call regarding my self-care was about to loom up. On this particular day the head nurse on my husband's unit called me into the nurse's office. "Sylvia, you are tired. I can see it in your eyes. Brian is fine and we are looking after him for you. You need a break." Oh my! Another learning curve looming! So, being by nature, one who would take bold steps in facing challenges head on – that was learned through life experiences – I found myself responding with "OK", I will make a promise to you. I will not visit for five days!" As I left her office, the impact of what I had just said hit home and my guts went into knots. Yes, I shed some tears on returning home but knew deep down that it was the correct thing to do. The up side to this would be that –

1. I got a much-needed rest and time to heal my emotional agenda
2. Brian would have a greater chance to finally settle in to his new home.

During those five days I decided to indulge in some "acceptance therapy" by getting rid of accumulated clutter plus set aside clothes to take to the care home for him.

Physical action can be a great emotional healer. I also made time to "go within" and tap into that universal peace and love, to gain strength for the ongoing journey. Surprisingly, the five days seemed to go quite quickly. Oh, by the way, I was also a good girl, and didn't call the care home as I knew that they would call me if there was an emergency. I am blessed that the care home is only about ten minutes drive away. I appreciate that for some folks you will have a bit of a journey for visiting and may have to schedule visits to fit in with your lifestyle. No matter where your loved is placed in care, you will have to face the reality of having made a choice to place your loved one in a place where you feel the care will be of a high standard. Yes, in certain cases there will be unexpected Care Home care required, for example after a situation having required hospitalisation, with discharge to their own home being impossible which then throws up a package of emotions. However, life is all about choices. Choosing to face challenges and seek to find blessings somewhere in the circumstances or become a long-term victim of the new circumstances.

Emotional extremes can influence how you behave when visiting your loved one. Either –

- Allowing guilt around having them placed into care, whereby you rush in to visit daily to check that they are OK and the staff are "up to standard" OR
- Not making an effort to visit at all and staying in denial so that you can avoid having to face up to what is happening.

From my personal journey perspective, visits were all about keeping my man as happy as possible along with maintaining as best a relationship as possible – maybe some fear also around him forgetting who I was fairly quickly?

It is important as carers, to try to put ourselves in their shoes, especially in the early days following admission to enable you to give of your very best to them, whilst also acknowledging your own needs. It is like a balancing act, walking a tight rope as it were. What do they do? Practice, Practice, Practice, to improve and perfect things.

CHAPTER 5

SELF-UNDERSTANDING AND CO-OPERATION

Suffice it to say that this journey as a carer cannot be "put in a box". All carers will be experiencing their own Alzheimer's Road. That being so, there are however, certain common emotional agendas that take place on this journey; It is my goal to help you face and deal with your emotions from a viewpoint of learning experiences to help with each stage of the journey and facilitate some amazing personal growth. You see, I do firmly believe, as I said earlier in choices in life and on a carers journey one has a choice as to how to deal with the challenges that come along. All experience can be a valuable lesson that we either learn from and search for the positive within it or stay in the victim mode mentioned earlier.

I can assure you that on my own journey to my husband's latter stage manifestations, I have been to the depths of despair and sorrow. My greatest help has come from the inner power that lies within us all that is waiting to give us a sense of inner calm and inner peace. Allowing that energy to help me face the changes and challenges head on. It has meant consistent practice of drawing on that inner strength and not allowing a victim mentality to lead the way.

I made a conscious decision early on when my husband had been admitted to Princess Christian to become friends with the staff. To work *with* them and encourage them in the great job they do. It takes special people to give from their heart twelve hours each day without showing any sign of frustration at repeated agitated and frustrated behavior from the residents. This is what happens in the Care Home, and I am truly grateful for love and friendship shown to the residents and also the relatives.

As a carer, it takes courage to choose to be an observer of what might really be going on when visiting rather than reacting to what you see at face value. Let me illustrate this for you –

Maybe like myself you have visited your loved one, only to find they are not shaved or properly dressed and hair looking unkempt. An immediate reaction could be to ask who did their personal care and why they are not properly dressed. Even wondering why they are just sitting in a chair and doing nothing. Having been "the other side of the fence" probably helps my approach, but my reaction would be and still is "he must have been challenging with personal care today and not wanting to join in activities!" OK, the staff have special training to deal with challenging behavior which will not mean that resident compliance is always going to happen. I know that with my husband, as with all the residents, they look for the best time to get maximum compliance with daily personal care and will try to encourage some degree of independence wherever possible. Sometimes when visiting on a "minimum compliance day" a carer will approach and say "Sorry, Brian is not shaved properly today, but it was difficult to get his co-operation". My response – "I gathered that when I arrived. It's OK, I know you are doing your best with his care and that at times it will be challenging for you." On a good day for him he is shaved, hair looking great and clothes wonderfully coordinated. In the earlier days they involved him in the choice of clothes, which was great as has always been a smart dresser with good colour coordination sense. One tactic used by one of the carers he had really bonded with, was to say to him "Brian, I have some lovely new clothes I would like you to try on for me" "Really!" would be his reply and immediately he would cooperate!

From a relative's perspective it is SO important that you give as much information as possible to the staff about your loved one to assist them in giving the very best standard of care possible. Of course, we must rule out the fact that as Alzheimer's neurons more and more kick in, then some past patterns of preferences may change. Let me illustrate – mentioned in the first book but no harm in repeating it for you.

For many years Brian was a coffee drinking man who had trained himself to indulge without sugar. He would drink coffee as his main drink each and every day. Imagine my surprise on an early admission visit, when I saw a carer making him a cup of tea with two sugars!! "Is this what he likes to drink?" I asked with a surprised voice "He's always been a coffee man". "Oh no! He now likes his tea plus two spoons of sugar!" was the response. What has also been interesting is that a drink of tea became a great distraction technique when I needed to leave, especially when he was manifesting agitation and angry frustration behaviour. I had more than likely stated on his admission his preference for coffee! Oh well, all part of the journey!

The more, as a carer, you can allow yourself to learn to be accepting of the day-to-day manifestations of the persons symptoms, as well as the changes, it will help you cope with the emotional part of your journey. How many times have I asked myself this question – "I wonder what is Really Going On in his brain and mind? How Aware Is He of what is now happening to him?" Maybe you ask similar questions as you try to sort it all out in your head. Let me share with you here that although I tell myself that there is no point in trying to figure it all out and just deal with each new bit of the journey as it manifests, I still have moments of wondering, especially when he has moments of complete clarity – more of that later.

The message I really want to get across is that to get the very best of care for your loved one means that a cooperative and understanding spirit with the care staff pays dividends. Yes, the cost of care seems almost crazy doesn't it? For me, I believe we need to do our part to help the staff give of their best to our loved one. How about noticing, for example, if a member of staff looks tired. Does it cost anything to ask if they are alright? They too are on their own day to day life journey – some many miles away from their home and family. Somehow, a little empathy and understanding seems to lift their spirit and you see new energy arising in them. Maybe if carers were more valued by visitors it would enhance their commitment to their career?

My husband has now been in Princess Christian Care Home for over three and a half years and I have watched some staff changes take place, but most of all, is the pleasure in sharing their progression from Carer to Senior Carer along with NVQ skills training progression. Recently I went to visit my husband and noticed that one of the male carers was no longer wearing a purple polo shirt but had a blue one on. "What's with the blue shirt?" I teased with a smile. His face lit up as he proudly told me he was now a senior carer and intended to progress all the way to NVQ level five! Wow! There's commitment from a guy who came all the way from the Asian continent with his brother to work at Princess Christian, worked hard on his English, as well as giving his all to the role of carer in a very challenging arena. He is one of many I have witnessed progressing from day one and rising to ranks of a new status.

Now let's continue some more with my own journey and the incredible learnings from it ......

CHAPTER 6

KEEPING A SENSE OF HUMOUR

Along with the money and house issue that kept arising in the early days, the next hurdle that appeared was the day that I visited after being brave enough to go five days without seeing my husband. As I drove to see him, I had mixed emotions going on. One was the excitement of seeing him, and the other was inner turmoil regarding what I would be facing. You may well be understanding this as you are reading! Yep! Still learning Sylvia, but looking back, I am grateful for the opportunity I have had to deal with my emotions and not let them rule my life. The more you are able to see emotional responses as something triggered from previous emotional events prior to the career journey – takes time to realise this – the more inner strength rises to acknowledge them and let them go, focusing on the good things in life and doing your best to bring that positive attitude to the caring journey.

So – on arrival at Princess Christian I took a deep breath, ignored the butterflies in my abdominal area, signed in the visitor's book to comply with fire regulations and proceeded to Bisley Unit. There he was relaxing in a chair and I excitedly went over to him ready to give him a big hug and a kiss when he gave me a look and angrily said "You've got another man haven't you!" Those words cut to my heart and I did my best to maintain a calm approach and then my best to reassure him it was definitely Not the case, that my commitment to him was 100%. He seemed to calm down and I stayed a good while before returning home. For the next few visits, I was greeted again and again "Are you sure you haven't got another man?" Gradually something seemed to register and it was not mentioned any more. As the early months progressed it became amusing to see him latching on to a particular lady and would often be walking around hand in hand with her when I arrived. Diplomacy being the best approach, I would greet Brian and tell the lady I had come to see my husband hoping it would make some sense to her. Brian would realise who I was and be happy to focus on his wife. From past times as a care home manager, I had witnessed "friendships" striking up with residents so was not surprised to watch his gregarious nature rising to the fore. Looking back, I recall the barn dancing days where he would pick a "particular" lady to demonstrate steps with and be positively subtly flirting with her! Not unusual then that he would respond to ladies in the unit who approached him. At least he was happy.

As the months progressed the "house" and "another man" were never mentioned any more. A relief for me, that made visiting easier with less "butterflies" to deal with. My confidence in the care he was receiving also helped greatly. I was always being kept up to date with how he was settling in with reassurance that he was happy most of the day. What a joy to be able to have peace about his care and sleep at night knowing he was in good hands and receiving high standard care.

The observational skills were amazing and I would be told if he had as much as a spot on his rear end – at home he was prone to boils in that area from time to time that responded well to homeopathic remedies and gradually lessened in frequency. Photographs were taken along with daily monitoring and updates reported to me when I visited.

Having been admitted primarily due to his aggressive "naughty neurons" behavior manifestation and major sundowning activity this was still the "norm" with him staying in the lounge most of the night.

My next learning curve was to maintain a sense of humour as I learned of two particular nocturnal escapades –

1. I had a phone call to tell me that on one of the regular checks during the night, somehow Brian had managed to get himself into one of the male residents rooms that was close by to his room. The staff observed him lying on the male resident's bed as we say "topping and tailing" with his head at the foot end of the bed and feet at the head end of the bed. Both were fast asleep and no harm was done! Understandably relatives have to be notified. I saw the amusing side of the incident and fortunately the other gentleman's relatives were not phased by what had happened. Never in a million years would my man have Ever shared a bed with another male!! He had very strong gender principles!!
2. This one involved a female resident but nothing more than an innocent occurrence! Brian was found sitting cross legged on the floor of her room and they were having a conversation of sorts! My response – "Well, at least he wasn't in bed with her!" It can happen of course if basic instincts kick in, but thankfully not with Brian.

From then on, I realised that being able to laugh at things was great therapy on the emotional roller coaster ride of the journey. Laughter, of course, releases positive, immune boosting chemicals into the blood stream. Much preferred over releasing those damaging stress hormones methinks!

A sense of humour was to bode well as his communication skills began to change and I had to do my level best to gauge what he was saying. How many times did I think he was wanting to go to the toilet?? Wrong!! "Don't be f…..g stupid! Of course, I don't" would be a very clearly spoken response. Yes, we went through a phase of the "F word becoming quite a prominent response with almost rehearsed regularity! All due to frustration at my not understanding the language being verbalized that was not matching his thoughts around what he wanted to express. Must have been so annoying for him. The most standard phrase I had thrown at me would be "What's the matter with you? Are you F…..g stupid or something?" I very quickly learned to reassure him about his challenge with knowing what he wanted to say and it not coming out in the right words in accordance to what he was thinking and the resulting misunderstanding by myself. Apologising for my not understanding seemed to help calm him. A sense of humour and patience are key mechanisms to surviving the carer journey. The understandable pain of watching someone slowly disappearing in front of you requires inner strength and courage and great fortitude to get through.

By now I was more and more drawing on my spiritual strength and using the peace mantra regularly as I knew from my personal development and coaching skills that repetition of positive statements Does Change Neuro Pathways. There is now scientific evidence with documented studies where neuron activity is recorded before and after the use of positive thinking mechanisms. Negative thought pathways change to positive, overriding the fear based way of thinking and living. So, the mantra for you to use is simple and easy to remember –

"I CHOOSE PEACE – ALL IS WELL IN MY WORLD"

SAY IT FREQUENTLY THROUGHOUT YOUR DAY AND MORE SO IN CHALLENEGING TIMES.

This doesn't mean life won't throw challenges your way anymore but a positive focus will enable you to tap into that place of deep inner peace and calm. As I stated earlier, I am still as I write, on my journey with my lovely husband and learning to operate from that place of inner calm and peace as the manifestations of his Alzheimer's change and the latter stages have kicked in. However, I made a decision that this journey would not totally consume me and neither would I become a victim of what was happening.

You too can find inner calm and peace if you choose to work at it. It lies deep within all of us. All you have to do is Stop, Breath, Say the Mantra, as you focus within your solar plexus (the belly) area for a few moments. Do it at least three times on rising and before sleep as a routine as well as recommended above.

CHAPTER 7

LOSING IT ALL DOWN THERE!!

My husband had always been a very particular man about his personal care and appearance.

I think back to the days when I was doing my subtle research before he was diagnosed and admit that the one thing I wanted to stay in denial about was the thought of him becoming doubly incontinent. The thought that he might even be aware of not being able to control his bladder, did not want to be faced if I am totally honest. Yet deep down I knew that one day I would have to face this actually happening.

On his admission to Princess Christian Care Home Brian was fully continent and just needed showing where the toilet was in his room for privacy. All was well it seemed, until I escorted him to the toilet whilst visiting him. He was beginning to show definite signs of cognitive and visual special impairment, along with obvious signs of increasing Posterior Cortex Atrophy symptoms. Insisting on still standing to empty his bladder, I had to stand clear as he "pointed percy" in the wrong direction creating a sizeable puddle on the floor to which he was quite oblivious. "Oh, that's better!" he would say. Discreetly I would guide him from the toilet doing my best to steer him clear of the puddle which was by now spreading and then report to a carer – they were well used to this with other residents as well as my man! At home I had managed to get him to sit on the toilet to relieve himself without any naughty neurons activity kicking in. He was definitely totally non-compliant with this now but at least he was totally unaware that he had missed the toilet pan! That gave peace of mind and acceptance of what I had initially dreaded would begin to happen prior to becoming fully incontinent. Yes, I was now on another acceptance phase on our journey and dealing with it with greater calm than expected. It is amazing how the mind can "predict" things to have a certain impact and then when the time comes it is not at all like imagined a while back. Acceptance in life is a great blessing if you flow with each moment and do not allow negative emotions to engulf you. I love a quote from a Reverend Michael Beckwith –

IT IS WHAT IS, ACCEPT IT
HARVEST THE GOOD
FORGIVE ALL THE REST

In my case it was - *Sylvia, accept where things are going now and be thankful that at least your man is unaware of what is happening every time he needs to empty his bladder. Then forgive yourself of any emotions that arise and be at peace.*

This journey is, in essence, a great opportunity to learn and release old emotional patterns and take each day and each moment as it comes. Don't fight the situation and project your own frustrations of things "not being normal" on to others. The clock cannot be turned back, and as a carer, you have to work at acceptance. Notice I said work at it. Yes, it does take effort. Nobody was more surprised than I was that the nursing and care management, coaching and a deep spiritual faith did not change the journey. How was I going to face it? Victim or Victor? I chose the latter and even as I write I am on another learning phase, a bit like being in a new classroom at college as new expressions of his disease are placed in front of me. One thing I appreciate is the support of my family and friends who remind me that I need to be mindful of balancing life.

A key tool used when visiting, because he still knows who I am, is to remind him of how much I love him and value his love plus how long we have been together without any major arguments. This cheers him up even if it only remains in his mind for a few moments. Expressing sincere feelings could bring up emotions of loss for me as I do this with each visit, but with practice I am now able to wear two hats as it were – his loving wife along with a more of a "carer" approach to the visit. Challenging moments are more easily dealt with from that "sense of humour" I talked about earlier. Especially when I am politely told that I am F.....g Stupid! I firmly believe that we have to work at this journey and not shy away from things that come up along the way. Life throws things at us anyway does it not? How you deal with life generally, may well reflect on how you deal with this journey.

It was a Tuesday afternoon for a pm visit and to possibly stay for supper. As I entered the lounge where he was sitting I could instantly see that all was not well with him. He was in very low spirits. I greeted him in my usual way and gave him a big hug. There was silence for a few moments and he then blurted out as he pointed to his lower regions "I think I am losing it all down there!" I took his hand in mine and lovingly looking at him asked "Do you really think so?" His short response was "Yes" and then he seemed not to want to discuss it any further yet was relieved to have shared it. Tea and cake was being served by now and that seemed to cheer him up and memory chats lifted his spirits a bit.

I spoke to the nurse before leaving, and yes, he was now beginning to be incontinent at times but refused to wear a pad or removed it after they had put it on. I suspected in my mind that somewhere in his mind he was still feeling as he used to and not considering the possibility of being incontinent. I never broached the subject again as it would be unkind to trigger further frustration and confusion moments. Like the day he flooded the conservatory lounge! As I entered, he was sitting on one of the sofas looking somewhat agitated. He suddenly went very pale and looked like he was going to faint on me! I called a carer who ran for the nurse. On checking his pulse, blood pressure and temperature, all seemed to be normal. Then the reason for him "taking a turn" was revealed. He suddenly stood up and as he did so urine poured through his trousers and on to the floor in a torrential rush. His bladder had filled to mega capacity causing momentary systemic shock until his neurons kicked in the message to have a pee. "Oh my" That feels better!" he joyously stated with a big smile on his face. Very diplomatically the carer took him away to change clothes and the floor was then thoroughly cleaned.

I now knew, for sure, it was time to accept a new part of his disease symptoms. It was actually a relief to me that he had been totally oblivious to emptying his bladder in an inappropriate place. It helped with my acknowledgement of things to myself without focusing negatively on the developments now occurring.

A few minutes later he appeared looking smart in a new pair of trousers and the visit continued as if nothing had happened – in his head nothing had happened out of the ordinary, had it? When sharing incidents like this one with my sister and close friend I did so with a sense of humour. It was best now, to be able to laugh at how he was behaving compared to what would have been his "norm". After all it is not Brian as we know and love him, it's those naughty neurons having more manifestation of messed up signals! A magazine that I used to reads over 30 years back, had a wonderful phrase that headed up a page of jokes – ***Laughter is the Best Medicine!***

Let's face it, it is good to keep a sense of humour around life situations is it not? Not to say you should never release through tears but not to get caught up in them permanently.

Sometimes I talk to myself – yes out loud too! "Sylvia, that's enough of that! Think of those happy memories!" I call it self-coaching and it works.

Have you got a photograph or something that will trigger a happy moment from the past? Put it where you can see it or hold it and re-live the experience with inner joy when those low times crop up with you. You will be amazed at how healing and uplifting it will be.

Before moving on I want to re-iterate how good the staff are at handling challenges with my husband, doing their very best to maintain dignity and a sense of self-worth. Keeping calm whilst doing their best to distract during times of agitation and frustration. His iPad is a great tool for that. Especially playing music.

CHAPTER 8

IT WOULD HAVE TO BE MY HUSBAND

I think back to my days as a care home manger plus working for a while as an agency staff nurse in the care home sector and can recall some "interesting" occurrences with residents who had some form of Dementia or Alzheimer's. There was the retired Bishop who led a very refined and Christian life where profanities were not part of his vocabulary. What a change with his dementia symptoms! Family had to speedily adjust to his new language skills filled with a great flow of profanities! Then there was the ex-army commander whose room was at the end of the corridor where the window looked out into the garden. Every evening he was escorted to his room and got ready for bed. Within a very short period of time he would appear from his bedroom complete with his bedding kit and set up camp below the window, making sure his "bed" was to military precision. There was no point in persuading him to return to bed as in his head he was on a military exercise where they slept out under the stars! Add in the male/female antics and you get the picture.

Now fast forward on my journey with my husband in Princess Christian where all the staff are excellent at keeping relatives informed of changes in behaviour etc., along with Brian's longstanding gregarious nature coming forward as he befriended female residents during the day time walking around hand in hand with them.

I witnessed this on more than one occasion during my visits. On this particular day as I approached the "happy couple" to say hello to my husband I felt constrained to deal with the what was happening very sensitively. I looked at the lady who was clutching his arm with determination to "own him" and politely said "Hello, Excuse me interrupting but I have come to see Brian who is my husband". I was immediately recognized with joy by Brian and as her husband had arrived to visit her at the same time, she reluctantly let go. Brian was oblivious to what had transpired and a happy time together was enjoyed on my visit. All part of the journey as residents will latch on to each other and maybe even think they are with their spouse as confused neurons express themselves.

That particular incident and other similar ones were of no consequence, but the day I was asked to go and see the nurse in the office was a different matter. I sensed the head nurse was aware it would be a sensitive issue to talk to me about as she took a breath and said "Sylvia, I have to tell you that we are allowing only male carers to deal with Brian's personal care now. He is touching up the girls breasts when they try to do things for him." My mind went back to those days when I witnessed things in my own care home and others I had worked in. Never dreaming it would take place with our journey. I couldn't help but smile and say to the nurse "On my!. It would have to be **my** husband!". A sense of humour saved the day here. There haven't been such incidents reported since, but his progression has manifested other personal care challenges. For whatever reason he reacts strongly to any personal care intervention. For a time it took maybe three staff to carry out his morning and evening routine care as his reaction was one of going absolutely rigid plus lashing out at the staff. As I write it takes two carers and he still reacts as before, and shouts and screams like a child not wishing to cooperate. To help alleviate the situation, his clothing has changed from smart trousers and shirt to joggers and polo shirts. He still gets as smart a pair of jogger type bottoms and colourful quality polo shirts albeit a size larger to minimize dressing and undressing challenges that benefits both Brian and the staff. However amazing they are at what they do for hm, I do have in mind their safety as well as my husbands – the team approach for best care of ones loved one.

For a good while following admission Brian continued to be a night owl wandering around until the early hours and being returned to his room to settle him or allow him to fall asleep in the chair in the lounge. Having had a chance to witness what goes on at night following a challenge discussed in a later chapter I am in awe of what the staff have to cope with during the night time hours. With dementia residents having a mixed up body clock there are always some that are up and about overnight behaving much as they do during the day time. Patience, and calm caring takes place as it does during the day. One lady I remember who was "on the go" all night still was "on the go" when I returned later in the day after a short sleep! "Where does she get her stamina? I could do with some of it!" I joked with the staff.

One other thing I observed overnight was something I had never seen anywhere else – even in my own care home due to company staffing policy. Something that in my estimation raised the home standards even higher. At around 5.30 am cleaners arrived to thoroughly clean the unit communal rooms, bathrooms and toilets to include removing chair cushions and almost spring cleaning with a special spray. Floors were washed with an antibacterial solution. The place smelt wonderful and was ready for the day time activity. Also, I have observed that each unit has its own dedicated cleaner who keeps all the rooms clean and sweet smelling and is always available for major spillages. The team of laundry staff work nonstop from morning to evening seven days a week and take great pride in their work.

As Brian's condition progressed further, night times began to change, and then another challenge arose to be faced by the staff and reported to me. He was now staying in bed at night but sleeping at the edge of the bed and tumbled out when he turned over. Thankfully no injury – he is made of tough stuff! He was then given a "low profile" bed that facilitated being lowered to the floor level along with a sensor mat on the floor. He continued to tumble out or he slept with half of him in the bed and the rest of him lay on the sensory mat. Of course, the efficiency of care, meant that very frequent reporting to me had to take place of the nocturnal escapades. The final remedy that has helped since is a standard bed with padded cot sides which I gave permission for. Now he was able to turn over and not fall out of bed. The other benefit was less phone calls to me!

Day time escapades then began to occur whereby he began to sit on a chair that wasn't there. By now his posterior cortex atrophy was becoming exacerbated even more and his risk of injury with falls needed to be managed. So, we increased the size of his trousers to accommodate hip protectors and they seemed to work. Life for me as the carer was certainly becoming more "interesting" with many phone calls about his daily falls but with no apparent injury sustained. One day I had one of those "aha moments". To save having to deal with the possibility of every mobile phone call being from the care home, I decided to invest in a low tariff phone that I called my care phone and gave the number to the staff. With a different ring tone, it saved me from that few seconds of what could be panic when the standard mobile phone rang. I would highly recommend this to generate at least some peace of mind on your journey. I managed to get a tariff for around five to six pounds a month which I figured was a worthwhile investment. Yes, you need to allow creativity to rise up as the journey progresses. Finding creative ways to deal with challenges will help with creating greater inner calm. All was going well with the falls strategies when –

It was around 7.45pm one evening and the care phone rang. Yes, he had fallen again but this time sustained a nasty cut over his right eye that was bleeding quite severely and required an ambulance to be called. They had literally just turned their back from checking the residents in the lounge he was in and then it happened. Just like young children, Alzheimer's residents can be safe one second and the very next second "it happens".

I stopped what I was doing and immediately left for the home – the blessing of living close by. When I arrived and entered the lounge, he was lying on the floor with his head supported with a pillow and one carer sitting on the floor with him to keep him calm and encouraging him to lie still whilst another carer was cleaning up a pool of blood on the floor. A short while later the ambulance crew arrived to assess the situation. They were incredible with the way they interacted with Brian and carried out basic observations. Taking his blood pressure along with carrying out a finger prick blood sugar levels triggered some shouting and a string of the "F" word that I hadn't heard for a while! On observing the cut it was decided that he ought to go to casualty for some suturing to be done. I began imagining an agitated, confused Alzheimer's patient in A & E as we wait for however long it takes to be seen whilst trying to keep him calm! I was now sitting with him to relieve the carer as it was the busy evening routine time. There was another option – send out a paramedic to put in a couple of stitches in the cut over the eye. Fortunately, this was arranged by the attending crew. They helped get Brian to sit in a chair – once again that "F" word echoed through the lounge! I sat with him until around midnight and was then advised by the night sister that I should go home and get some sleep as they could manage him.

When I returned the next morning, I was informed that the paramedic had arrived at around 4am and used steri-strip dressings to bring the cut together. I'm sure this was a challenge for Brian and a few more interesting behaviours took place! Well, he was in great spirits and seemed oblivious to the dressing over his eye and showing no sign of pain or discomfort – we would know if he was in pain as he has a very low pain threshold!

As I share my journey with you, I want you to get a feel for my ongoing learning to tap into that inner calm as often as possible and to "stay in the moment". Accepting the changes in how the disease manifests. It takes practice to stay loving and caring without allowing emotions to consume you or to project them on to others who are doing their utmost to give wonderful care.

As each stage of the disease manifests new challenges, it is important to learn to accept the changes and work at acknowledging even the smallest of positives. In a world full of fear and stress where the negative tales seem to be top priority, it takes fortitude to decide to find a piece of joy in each day, but with practice it is possible. Even waking up each day to say – I CHOOSE TO CREATE JOYOUS MOMENTS THIS AND EVERY DAY

Then add in the peace mantra – I CHOOSE PEACE, ALL IS WELL IN MY WORLD

I challenge you to do this. It will not only help you as a carer but will have assured health benefits as you release immune system supporting chemicals into the blood stream. That is what positive thoughts and words create and is now proven by science. Let's face it, you need to look after You to successfully ride the emotional roller coaster journey. It is all about choice, as is life in general –

Will you be a Victim of Circumstances OR be an Overcomer of Circumstances?

CHAPTER 9

FOOD GLORIOUS FOOD

My husband has always had a wonderful appetite and never been fussy with his food. I have always said that he has hollow legs that we fill up first and then his stomach! It was certainly a blessing when I became wheat and dairy intolerant as I could create wheat and dairy free meals and he would tuck in with great relish! Probably enhanced his health too as a side benefit. His appetite trend has not changed on his Alzheimer journey to date. He seems to like coffee or green tea with honey for breakfast and then move to his tea with two sugars.

On his admission to Princess Christian, he was able to feed himself and take drinks when offered. He was also no problem with taking medication with a drink. He soon became known by all for his veracious appetite for food. No issue with him getting daily nutrition from his diet! Breakfast was the same as at home and remains the same – porridge with molasses and a tablespoon of coconut oil and MCT oil for helping brain tissue (Dr Mary Newport). The care staff still continue this ritual for him. It is a superb tool for gaining initial morning cooperation with him. They certainly have creative skills with the residents! As relatives, as said earlier, you can certainly help with care by providing little character and preference traits on admission and as time passes if you suddenly remember something and feel good about assisting with gaining quality care levels. It's the little traits and habits that can be key to gaining there compliance when needed.

On my husband's admission I completed a very comprehensive form for his file that assisted in his daily care. Knowing particular challenges taking place was also a key part of the information. This would of course change as time went on and they would be informing me of changing behaviours! With Brian it was important for them to know his cognition levels and the typical Posterior Cortex Atrophy traits as contrasting colours were important – at home I had changed to contrasting red and white crockery and red handled cutlery to enable independence as long as possible.

Your journey will be assisted with you realising the power of acceptance as you journey.

As time went on, he started to have difficulty with using cutlery and recognizing where the food was on his plate. Mealtimes became interesting to observe when I had meals with him. As with personal care, he still had an awareness that he should be able to do things for himself and frustration kicked in at the meal table "Look at That! Did you see that?" he would angrily shout as yet another portion of his meal shot to the floor. Sometimes there would be more food on the floor than his plate! "Let me help you darling" I lovingly suggested one day. Oops! Mistake as he retorted back to me "F... off! I can do it!". It took time for him to allow assistance from the staff and a subtle application of a plate guard to be applied to help him. General observation as a visitor challenged with acceptance of disease progress, could easily be "Why are they not helping him with his food?". Maybe, like my husband, they are not ready to let go and allow others to help as they still believe they can do everything for themselves. Boy, do you have to learn the secret of adapting to change! When you do it will help you cope better. Always visiting without a fixed agenda and pre-conceived ideas. Also being in their world always will help with preventing upset and arguments. If they think you are someone else in a particular moment then be that person with them. Next time they may well know who you are.

Are you someone who worries about the future or pre-empts what could happen? That was me years ago and then I had one of those light bulb moments – it never turned out quite as I had imagined! That enlightening has been a wonderful asset to visits, keeping a flexible approach to what one will be faced with and not to take everything at face value but seek to see behind what is being shown in both words and behaviour.

Mark Twain comes to mind here –

I HAVE HAD MANY WORRIES IN MY LIFE; MOST OF WHICH NEVER HAPPENED

So, back to "food glorious food". During the first eighteen months following admission Brian happily went on outings to garden centres and cafés for morning coffee and cakes. My lifestyle meant that I could accompany him on many of the trips plus help with wheelchair pushing as needed. It wasn't long before Brian was known as the "helper" at the table. Drinks and cakes were ordered and served to all. Usually there would be maybe two or three fairy cakes left over which were offered around for a second indulgence. Most refused and then came the standard question "Brian, would you like another cake? There are a couple left and we don't want to waste them, do we?" "Ooh! Yes please!" as eyes lit up, he always replied and then tucked in with all speed to the remaining cakes. Relatives and helpers all knew what would happen with those left-overs but it became part of the fun of the outings.

Now for the exciting part. By the time we returned lunch had begun. Yes, you have guessed it. He then indulged in his normal lunch and pudding portions, with a second portion of pudding sometimes!

As time progressed, the staff, with the greatest of patience and skill on their part, succeeded in gaining Brian's approval for help with his meals. When I visited it was a different story. It was if his neurons reverted back to when he was at home with me, being able to do things for himself. He would get angry and confused. I had the sense to call a staff member to assist him and allay further agitation. "I'm sorry guys" I would say "Can you help Brian as he won't let me assist him". They came to help him every time I asked and he was 100% accepting of their interaction. With drinks he could manage for a long time, so long as they were given to hold with two hands along with a bright coloured drinking vessel to help with object recognition and facilitate increased sensory touch skills. It is so important to give the person some sense of being in control, if at all possible, within the restraints of their safety and as their loved one, comes to terms with any dietary intervention that may be necessary. So much has been learned during his time in 24/7 care about balancing what I have known about his innate preferences around food and drink with how the Alzheimer's neuron activity can influence best practice for overall quality of care.

I have watched my man travel from being able to manage independently with food and drink, progress to requiring thickened drinks and a soft diet to aid with swallowing. I recently had another learning curve on this one. I was feeding Brian with chopped up breaded chicken pieces along with vegetables and curly fries that had gravy with them to soften when he suddenly began to choke and change colour. He was fairly upright in his chair but obviously needed to be sitting as high as possible. Staff intervened and then he was brought a very soft diet that included mashed potatoes. Understandably it gave him a real fright – and I was somewhat distressed. "Definitely totally soft diet from now on, eh?" I said to the nurse. "He has to be fully upright for eating plus only very small amounts at a time now" I was kindly told. What did I learn from this? Primarily not to feel guilty about the incident and to be mindful of where he now is on this journey when I am feeding him. It was not long before he was enjoying his new lunch followed by soft chocolate sponge and custard that slipped down with ease. His love of food will override the need for soft foods. They will still taste good to him.

You cannot bring back what was, so one might as well take each moment as it comes as I have stated earlier without guilt, denial or fear. We can never turn back the clock can we? What is happening right this moment will become history in a second. Don't allow the past to influence the future.

Look ahead with a knowing, that, as I say – "Everything is in Divine order" with a choice of having your cup half full or half empty.

A bit of a pun there after the food and drink!

CHAPTER 10

BE READY FOR SUPRISES!

My husband's hobbies revolved around music. Since his teens he was involved in the folk world and had voice training which resulted in him having a lovely singing voice. Over the years he was an active member of a folk club in his home area of Cambridge. When he moved to Surrey, he then joined and became very active in the Dorking Folk Club. He was a popular "floor singer" in many folk clubs in the south east. From this background had emerged an interest in folk and barn dancing resulting in him forming his own band called Stockbrokers Belt based in Surrey – very aptly named with many wealthy people living in the county. He was not an avid reader, although he did collect many books, mainly historical and informative or linked to his folk singing. He also was involved in local radio becoming a regular participant in some programs, becoming friends with some of the DJ's and going into the local studio from time to time.

So here he was in Princess Christian Care Home with a very niche set of interests – not having possessed a television, he would not be familiar with popular programs unless visiting family and friends. This was a bit of a challenge for the activities team apart from the regular musical entertainment. He really got into this with feet tapping. Clapping, whooping and whistling. In the early days he would join in the singing of songs he could recall.

One morning I called in to see him as the head of activities was attempting to get him to join in things. "Hello Brian" her cheery voice called out "How are you today? We are going to make some cakes today. Would you like to join us?". His face said it all! "No thank you" was the stern reply. So I chipped in with "cooking was never one of his favourite pastimes" and laughed. A cup of tea with two sugars and biscuits was more up his street at 11am!

I couldn't help reminiscing on my own experience in the care home I was managing that helped me appreciate the challenges the activity team have each day to do their very best to get residents to participate in different activities.

One day in particular stands out when the area manager visited "why aren't the residents doing activities?" was the almost angry question. Knowing the dedicated effort our activities organizer put in, I was determined to get a message across "Patty works very hard to create different activities based on the residents' interests" I replied "However, many of them refuse to get involved" Yes, this is true that the mood of the day will affect interest in taking part. Of course, there are those that are up for anything and join in most days whereas others will absolutely dig their heels in and would rather just sit around all day long. In the Dementia/Alzheimer's arena the key to hopefully gaining interest is to tap into past interests. The iPad memory tool is great for this with one-to-one interaction and also help stimulate those neurons. Especially in the mid to latter stages.

Remember my husband and his very niche past interests I told you about? Well, I am now about to spring a surprise on you!

One morning I arrived for one of my regular visits, to be greeted by a member of staff who joyously informed me that Brian was enjoying a game of Bingo. "What? You are kidding me!" was my very shocked response "He hates Bingo and has never played it in his life! His first wife's addiction to Bingo set the stage for him Never to get involved with it and overtly decry it to others!"

As I entered Bisley Unit, there he was sitting with a carer to assist marking off his numbers. I took her place and continued to help mark off the numbers with him. He completed a line and I shouted "Bingo!". It was at that moment I realised why he might decide to join in – his prize was chocolate! He loved chocolate and chocolate sweets. I am convinced the thought of winning chocolate encouraged him to take part.

So when you get concerned that your loved one is not joining in with activities, don't despair. Remember that old saying – *You can lead a horse to water but you can't make it drink?* I occasionally add another bit to it – *Sometimes you can't even take a horse to the water!"*

When there were outings scheduled, Brian did enjoy going on those for his tea/coffee and cakes that are all a part of it. The minibus ride could be a little challenging but was dealt with calmly. I went with him to a *coffee and concert morning at Guildford Cathedral* and he was not overly happy on that day but didn't decline coming with us. The singer was indulging us in light operatics and Brian was showing signs of absolute boredom. I was hoping he wouldn't shout out something rude about the singing but was saved from concern when she began to sing a popular folk song. "She's singing one of my songs!" declared Brian and immediately sat upright and was joining in! That moment was discussed avidly as soon as the concert finished to facilitate a calm return journey.

This journey is full of surprises and you never know when a special moment is going to occur. Never pre-judge things as I said earlier and try to work it all out in your head because you won't!

When visiting you can always ask for your loved one's memory pad to help with creating a good time with them – hopefully! This is where Princess Christian scores well having invested in having reminiscence iPads for the residents. Yes, you need to be involved and supply the photographs, music ideas etc. but it will pay off in the long run. I will often ask for my husband's iPad and play music and sing the songs to him – if he is in the mood. It certainly helps if you are stuck with what to talk about. OK, I have asked him if he would like to listen to music after Sunday lunch to be very gruffly told "No Thank You!" That triggers me to just sit with him for a while until he seems to be tired and falls asleep full of the lovely roast lunch and trifle.

Just sitting with your loved one can be important as they may at some level be aware of your presence and be comforted by it.

Where he is at on his journey now you really have to grab those moments when he is alert and alive because sometimes you will get a surprise spell of absolute clarity about something. Somehow the neurons connected somewhere along the line. Angry frustrated ones also kick in and that's alright. After all we all have those "off days" don't we?

With a large garden available to sit in and benches out at the front of the home that catch the sun make it possible to indulge in fresh air from time to time. Hmm, another surprise here.

Previously Brian had not been totally disinclined to being in the outdoors and we would go to the coastal towns for the day in the warmer weather and walk along the canal path as we were very close to the Basingstoke Canal. So I decided to take him outside for some sun and fresh air after lunch one day. There was a bit of a breeze but it was lovely and warm. I made sure he had a jumper on and off we went. As soon as I got him outside in the sun a gentle breeze blew "It's cold!" he declared. I managed to get him to sit on one of the benches for a few minutes but he repeated that he was cold. "Do you want to go back in then?" I decide to ask. "Yes!" was the curt response. It's interesting how sometimes the please and thank can also disappear sometimes when it was programmed way back in childhood. No big deal though!

One thing I have noticed with my man is that, in amongst his aggressive agitated moments when things need to be done for him, he is very often showing gratitude especially around drinks and food. Give him a drink of tea and he will say "That's lovely" with a big smile. Tell him tea and cakes are coming soon and face lights up "Ooh Really!" is the excited reaction! One can see what a major distractive tool his food and drink can be. Everyone will have their unique something to try to distract from agitation and frustration expression.

If you think about it, as a carer you are also going to have your own moments of frustration. So let me remind you of the very powerful mantra again –

I CHOOSE PEACE
ALL IS WELL IN MY WORLD

CHAPTER 11

THE DUMMY RUN AND IT'S OUTCOMES

It was a typical Sunday morning and I was looking forward to lunch with my husband as usual. His mood changes made no difference to my dedication of time with him. I had learned when to stay and when to walk away or interact with other residents and then go back to him. He would think I had just arrived.

Unless I had to go away on life purpose activity or was taking a break to care for me, Sundays with him had become a weekly ritual that I enjoyed as usually there were at least some moments of laughter and fun with him to remember. iPhone always being to hand to capture special moments as a photograph or video. When my fiend visits from Lincolnshire her video skills come into play and I now possess some great footage to put together as a film for memories to look back on and share with those who love him.

The relationship with the staff was such that if I had to skip a few of my regular days I would be greeted with "Are you alright? Where have you been? We missed you!" That is how much of a family environment is created in the care home. And I can honestly say that my response is usually "It's good to be back!"

This particular Sunday was in November of 2017 and when I entered the unit, I could not see him in any of the lounges so assumed he had been late complying with getting up and dressed. I spoke to one of the carers who immediately directed me to the nurse in charge. I knew then that there might be more things than my initial thought. Then the news broke "Sylvia, Brian had a seizure whilst being showered this morning so we have put him back to bed. This can happen in the later stages of Alzheimer's Disease. Other residents have had a sudden seizure and then been absolutely fine" Relieved to hear that I went to his room where he was resting and looked tired from what had occurred. I touched and spoke quietly to him as he may also have been administered a mild sedative to help calm the brain activity. As I sat with him, suddenly his colour changed and he began to violently convulse. I pressed the emergency button and ran for a carer or nurse. Their response was immediate plus they rang for an ambulance as he was beyond simple measures of management. My nursing background told me that this could be life threatening and was followed by my own manifestation of shock as the possibility of a traumatic way of leaving this earth had not ever crossed my mind. The ambulance crew carried out immediate emergency measures and prepared for him to be taken to the nearest Accident & Emergency Department. I called my sister in Scotland and requested a prayer chain to be started for him. Blessed to have the support of friends close by I then phoned one who had always said she could be called at any time day or night if I needed anything. Amazingly she was at home and immediately left everything to come to the care home and drove me to the hospital as a follow on to the ambulance. Also, it was a blessing that his longstanding favourite carer was on duty. He went as an escort with Brian in the ambulance. It was also him who had done his very best for Brian with his first seizure. He was probably going through his own shock also, no matter how well trained! He told me later that evening how he felt he should have been able to do more. I reassured him that he must have done a superb job as he had managed to get Brian to the floor without further injury.

As my friend drove, I worked on my inner peace skills in amongst allowing my shock to be released. The carers had grown very fond of Brian and a few had tears in their eyes I noticed the next morning and another favourite carer of his was genuinely upset and I gave him a hug. It is important to remember that the professional carers also have their own emotions and feelings to deal with as they cannot help but bond with residents – that is what enhances care standards. They need support as much as we do.

On arrival at the hospital, we were told to wait until they had got him into a cubicle. After what seemed a long wait, we were ushered through to the CPR unit – where it is touch and go as to whether he will make it. In full swing were monitors, intravenous sedatives as well as oxygen being given. There, he had at least three further seizures, and as advised by my friend who is a spiritual minister, I spoke to Brian and gave him permission to walk through the door from this world to the next. It would be cruel to hold him here to go through major suffering if it was his time to leave. As we sat in the waiting room the doctor informed me that he was keen to admit my man for a week and do tests and scans to find a cause for the seizures. I firmly refused this and told him all that was required was for Brian to be kept comfortable without further intervention and that I wished for him to return to the care home as soon as was possible. I went back to sit with him as he was now in another cubicle and stable.

Then what I can only describe as miracles took place.

1. Princess Christian agreed to care for him if all relevant medication could be there for him.

2. A lovely elderly care physician appeared to see Brian and stated "He is definitely going home." Here is not the place for him. I will organize all his drugs for him and if necessary, I will arrange for them to be delivered by courier to the care home. Wait here, I will be back." She then got the on-call pharmacist to come in and sort out all the required drugs which were couriered to the care home and we eventually returned at around 11pm. My good friend had taken back the carer and returned home as I accompanied my man in the ambulance.

The casualty staff were indeed amazing and the overall care superb while we were there.

I stayed the night with Brian and he went into a deep sleep but with noticeable breathing changes. He survived the night and was "hanging in there" on the Monday morning.

The lovely care home manager came and asked if I would like the last rights to be served. I agreed and it seemed to bring a great sense of peace into his room. Well, I do believe in ministering angels. There must have been some sent to us! His favourite cousin and husband came up plus my best friend from Lincolnshire arrived to support and stay a while as she bonded well with him. Once again, a blessing amongst the anguish. It was still a bit of touch and go for a few days more.

Now here are the next amazing outcome folks! On the Monday – the day of the last rights, the hospice nurse was supposed to come and insert a syringe driver with continuous sedatives to be administered as he was not expected to make it. They didn't turn up!

By the end of the week, he was taking fluids and a pureed diet, had returned to how he had been prior to the seizures AND with some increased communication and cognition skills!

The next visit from cousin and husband left them absolutely astounded at how he was interacting. It was mid-December; my sister was visiting to stay over the Christmas period so the staff had organized a tea party for us complete with a decorated trolley adorned with posh cups and saucers – mug for Brian of course - teapot and milk jug. We had a great time together with Brian stringing sentences together and smiling and laughing!!What a memory eh?

Yes, I did have an emotional outburst with the receptionist and housekeeper on the Monday when we thought he might not make it which taught me to acknowledge my grief and express it, but I did not allow it to linger and take hold with fear of the future. A decision to value every moment I spend with Brian was made on that day and stills stands.

He has had no further seizures. Sedation was gradually reduced and usual medication continued with one dose of diazepam at night.

In spite of being in the late stages of Alzheimer's with full care in all aspects, he still recognizes me on every visit and we enjoy a few minutes of a sort of conversation and laughter.

One interesting thing I am observing when I visit is that he seems to have recovered ability to retain small amounts of information plus has clarity about what I am communicating to him. For example, I was telling him of a pending visit from my sister and this was not the first mention of it. "Maureen will be down to visit again in a couple of weeks" I said to him. "I know" was his response. Almost as if he had remembered what I had said previously. This has happened also with the visits from my good friend from Lincolnshire. He also fully understood about up-to-date things I have been talking about – "Yesterday was the trooping of the colour. The queen was in a carriage as she is 92 years old now". His response "Really!" about the queens age, with a smile on his face. The following day – roast lunch day he also fully got it when I told him that it was Prince Phillips 97th birthday and that he was no longer carrying out official duties. Then when I told him it was roast lamb for lunch, he through his hands up in the air with a "Wow! Great!" excited response. He may not have got So excited in the past but he knew exactly what I was telling him to be able to thus respond.

I have also noticed with him that he seems to catch conversation close by and will add a comment, maybe just one word, but he has not missed what was being said and at some level understand what is being said.

Why am I sharing this? Because I firmly believe that we never know when someone with either Alzheimer's Disease or a form of Dementia, somewhere within the muddled neurons, actually does hear, with some degree of understanding, what is being said. Thus said, let me also mention that it would make sense therefore, not to "talk over" your loved one when visiting. Even if they seem to be semi-sleeping or in another "zone". I recall my nursing days when it was drummed into us that hearing is the last sense to go so, we were NEVER to talk over patients who were dying or in a coma.

Because we are still trying to more fully understand the brain and dementia disease expression, from my observations, we need to be sensitive with "conversation" as they may understand more than we give them credit for. Maybe also it is worth mentioning here that **What** we talk about may also need to be considered to prevent upset and agitation from observing how visits go –

Another recent episode with my husband occurred when I turned up to visit with a cake for him that had been lovingly made by a friend, we had both known for some years but he had not seen since his early onset period. "Hey Brian, I have a lovely homemade cake here for you from the lady who runs Walton Church." "Ooh lovely!" he said with a big smile.

"Remember when we used to go there together? It was in a church that we met, wasn't it?" I continued. The cake was served with his afternoon mug of tea and went down with a smile of gratitude. "We are blessed with all our friends, aren't we?" I said as we sat quietly together. "Yes" he replied but was looking a bit sad. Head looking down he suddenly sighed" Oh, Crikey." And I felt that he knew what was going on with his Alzheimer's in that moment. I hugged him "It is hard, isn't it?" "Yes" was his answer, as he almost welled up with tears. Then I found myself responding with "I do try to understand what it is like for you darling" and just sat quietly with him. He then seemed to drift off as if tired and I slipped away to go home.

That did impact on me for a while and taught yet more about not preempting anything on the carers journey. We cannot really know fully what is happening within their thought processes in amongst the confusion.

Speaking of preempting things – as in life generally – I am smiling as I tell you more of our journey.

It is now 2018 and with how things were progressing I had been thinking that he would not get through 2016, and then 2017. Here we are, following a major incident that was in essence a "dummy run", still journeying with a dear man with some seeming clarity and ability to understand conversation, albeit he can do nothing for himself!

Well, Well! All I feel I need to re-iterate as we draw to a close now is –

- Don't assume anything on your journey but know that you Can have moments that are truly positive. Be ready to face surprises, keep a sense of humour throughout AND remember to take care of you.
- Remember to value and appreciate the care staff who are doing the very best they can for your loved one. The more you build rapport and understanding with them, you will travel the 24/7 care road with a greater understanding of yourself and others also involved.
- Tap into the inner peace daily for every aspect of your care journey and life in general.
- Remember that there is choice in everything to be a victim or a Victor!

CHAPTER 12

A SUMMARY OF LITTLE TIPS

This book has primarily been about the emotional aspect of the 24/7 care journey.

There are organisations available to help with funding issues, how to find a "five star" care home in terms of quality of care. A simple and basic environment that meets the required standards and has ongoing innovative ideas with dedicated staff, who care from the heart, far outweighs a five-star hotel like appearance that does not offer five-star care.

The power of the internet is phenomenal now with many organisations ready to help.

Facing 24/7 care in a care home can be very positive. It is definitely not a sign of your personal failure. I realised that on my own journey and have become part of another family, enjoying being involved with the Friends of Princess Christian Care Home, supporting the home where I can. Getting involved really can help you on your journey.

Here are a few summary tips –

- Don't be afraid of facing 24/7 Care Home Care. There are some amazing ones out there
- Accept that there may be some settling in hurdles to overcome
- Give as much information about your loved one as possible. More information = better care for your loved one
- Build a rapport with the staff
- Stand back and observe the whole picture and don't pre-judge on face value
- Appreciate the staff whenever you can – we all thrive on praise, don't we?
- Remember to care for You and take a break. We have the power of Skype and other online communications now to stay in touch

ABOUT THE AUTHOR

Sylvia has developed a passion for supporting the emotional perspective of journeying as a Dementia Carer. Her varied nursing career, care management and running Care Home became invaluable when her husband was diagnosed with Young Onset Alzheimer's Disease. From childhood she had a deep reliance on God that carried her through the tough times in her life. In spite of her experiences and spiritual faith, this journey had to be taken! Sylvia is keen to help others ride "The Emotional Roller Coaster" of caring.

MORE PUBLICATIONS BY SYLVIA

- *The Rocky Road of Naughty Neurons*

- *Riding The Emotional Roller Coaster*

- *Sylvia's Little Book of Emotional Quotes*

- *From There to Here, Journey of a Skinned Rabbit*

- *Video Tips volumes One Two and Three*

AVAILABLE AT AMAZON

WEBSITE: https://dementia-whisperer.com
FACEBOOK: https://www.facebook.com/alzheimerskeepitpositive
TWITTER: https://twitter.com/bryden_stock/

Email: info@dementia-whisperer.com

www.ingramcontent.com/pod-product-compliance
Lightning Source LLC
LaVergne TN
LVHW040157080526
838202LV00042B/3201